TABLE OF CONTENTS

1.0 INTRODUCTION 1
2.0 TRAINING STRATEGIES 5
   2.1 Bad Cardio vs. Good Cardio 6
   2.2 Body Part Isolation vs. Complex Movements in Strength Training 9
   2.3 Tired of the Same Old 3 Sets of 10? So is Your Body! Discover How to Manipulate Training Variables 11
   2.4 Your Workouts Need Both Consistency and Variability for Max Results 13
   2.5 The Ultimate Hard-Body Exercise 15
   2.6 Barbell, Kettlebell, and Dumbbell Complexes - a Different Style of Weight Training for a Ripped Body 18
   2.7 Top 15 Non-Traditional, Muscle-Building, Fat Blasting Workouts! 22
3.0 NUTRITION STRATEGIES 31
   3.1 Post-Workout Nutrition: Secrets to a Hard, Lean Body 32
   3.2 Don't be Afraid of Dietary Fat! Even Some Saturated Fats are Healthy for You 34
   3.3 Healthy Trans Fats vs. Unhealthy Trans Fats Revealed 42
   3.4 The Top Fitness Foods to Stock Your Cabinets With…Making Smart Choices Starts at the Grocery Store 45
   3.5 Are Vitamin/Mineral Supplements Necessary or Just Money Down the Toilet? 51
   3.6 Make Healthier Choices When Forced to Eat Fast-Food 54

1.0 INTRODUCTION

Inside this book, you're going to find various powerful strategies to make your training and nutrition program more exciting and result producing. You'll find out the truth about cardio. You'll discover some extremely effective strength training exercises, tips, and strategies. You'll even discover some new training styles that have emerged in recent years as well as some fresh ideas you've probably never thought of before. I'll also give you some great healthy meal ideas and unbiased nutritional strategies…none of that low-carb or low-fat gimmicky crap! I'm also NOT going to give you any of the same old BS that you've heard from mainstream health professionals about how you need to do endless hours of boring cardio routines, and eat nothing but bland meals like tuna and rice, or plain grilled chicken with broccoli in order to get in great shape. HELL NO!

Instead, I'm going to show you that you can enjoy life to the fullest while simultaneously building the body of your dreams and increasing your energy so that you feel like a million bucks every single day. Not only that, but you'll be able to perform like never before…whether it's performing physical tasks at home, dominating the competition on the playing field, or even performing in the bedroom! Yes, these are all just the start of some of the benefits of striving to achieve your own peak fitness.

Aside from the fact that you can take action now and improve how you look, feel, and perform, one of the most important aspects of taking responsibility for your own fitness is that you'll live a longer, happier life and reduce your risk of degenerative diseases. In all seriousness, the health condition of the majority of people in developed nations has deteriorated to such an extent that it has literally become a crisis. In the US, experts estimate that approximately 70% of the adult population is currently overweight or obese. That means that if you are a lean and healthy individual, you are a minority! It has literally become the norm for most people to be out of shape, overweight, and ridden with degenerative diseases like type-II diabetes, heart disease, and cancer. That's pretty sad. With as fast as obesity rates are increasing, if things don't change soon, we could very likely see 9 out of every 10 people as overweight or obese in another decade or two.

Something needs to give. People need to start taking responsibility for their own health and fitness and that of their families. Nobody else is going to do it. The billion dollar food manufacturing companies sure aren't going to do it. All they want to do is make huge profits by selling you cheap junk food, heavily refined and processed full of chemicals that are causing a cellular disaster within your body. The billion dollar pharmaceutical companies sure aren't going to look out for your health either. Hell, they want you to be sicker than ever, so that you'll have to buy more of their medicines. And the rich supplement companies won't look out for your health either. They love the fact that people are getting fatter all the time, so that they can persuade you with fancy marketing into thinking that there's a quick-fix solution and all you have to do is spend lots of money on some of their pills and you'll magically be lean and mean without changing anything else in your life.

It's pretty simple as to why the world is becoming a fatter place at an astonishing rate. For one, the population has become increasingly more sedentary over the years. Kids no longer spend most of their time running around and playing games outside. Now, they spend more time inside playing video games or surfing the web on the computer. Adults do less manual labor than ever before. Technology allows us to be lazier than ever and perform as little movement as we want on a daily basis. This simply means that we must intentionally add extra movement to our daily lives in this day and age where we're not required to do much movement any more. My thinking is…why does it have to be a chore to add movement to your daily life? It should be the opposite…you should be active because you enjoy it! For example, if you're not the least bit interested in weight training, then find something you do like such as swimming, rock climbing, mountain biking, or competitive sports, and enjoy it on a regular basis.

Another reason the world is becoming fatter is that our food supply has become more heavily processed, refined, filled with chemicals, and modified from its natural state over the years. Everybody thinks that they don't have time in this fast-paced world to prepare their own meals anymore, so they grab quick junk foods from corner stores, fast food joints, and restaurants. This habit makes it that much harder to stay healthy and lean, because THEY aren't looking out for your health. Only YOU can do that!

The solution is easy! First, we need to make smart whole food decisions, and prepare our own meals. Second, we need to get out and move. Our bodies are meant to move and be active on a regular basis. That's the simplest way to look at it. Now let's get down to some of the insider secrets from a fitness junkie on how you can get top notch results out of both your training and your nutrition programs.

2.0 TRAINING STRATEGIES

2.1 Bad Cardio vs. Good Cardio

It is common to hear fitness professionals and medical doctors prescribe low to moderate intensity aerobic training (cardio) to people who are trying to prevent heart disease or lose weight. Most often, the recommendations constitute something along the lines of "perform 30-60 minutes of steady pace cardio 3-5 times per week maintaining your heart rate at a moderate level". Before you just give in to this popular belief and become the "hamster on the wheel" doing endless hours of boring cardio, I'd like you to consider some recent scientific research that indicates that steady pace endurance cardio work may not be all it's cracked up to be.

First, realize that our bodies are designed to perform physical activity in bursts of exertion followed by recovery, or stop-and-go movement instead of steady state movement. Recent research is suggesting that physical variability is one of the most important aspects to consider in your training. This tendency can be seen throughout nature as animals almost always demonstrate stop-and-go motion instead of steady state motion. In fact, humans are the only creatures in nature that attempt to do "endurance" type physical activities. Most competitive sports (with the exception of endurance running or cycling) are also based on stop-and-go movement or short bursts of exertion followed by recovery. To examine an example of the different effects of endurance or steady state training versus stop-and-go training, consider the physiques of marathoners versus sprinters. Most sprinters carry a physique that is very lean, muscular, and powerful looking, while the typical dedicated marathoner is more often emaciated and sickly looking. Now which would you rather resemble?

Another factor to keep in mind regarding the benefits of physical variability is the internal effect of various forms of exercise on our body. Scientists have known that excessive steady state endurance exercise (different for everyone, but sometimes defined as greater than 60 minutes per session most days of the week) increases free radical production in the body, can degenerate joints, reduces immune function, causes muscle wasting, and can cause a pro-inflammatory response in the body that can potentially lead to chronic diseases. On the other hand, highly variable cyclic training has been linked to increased anti-oxidant production in the body and an anti-inflammatory response, a more efficient nitric oxide response (which can encourage a healthy cardiovascular system), and an increased metabolic rate response (which can assist with weight loss). Furthermore, steady state endurance training only trains the heart at one specific heart rate range and doesn't train it to respond to various every day stressors. On the other hand, highly variable cyclic training teaches the heart to respond to and recover from a variety of demands making it less likely to fail when you need it. Think about it this way -- Exercise that trains your heart to rapidly increase and rapidly decrease will make your heart more capable of handling everyday stress. Stress can cause your blood pressure and heart rate to increase rapidly. Steady state jogging and other endurance training does not train your heart to be able to handle rapid changes in heart rate or blood pressure. Steady state exercise only trains the heart at one specific heart rate, so you don't get the benefit of training your entire heart rate range.

The important aspect of variable cyclic training that makes it superior over steady state cardio is the recovery period in between bursts of exertion. That recovery period is crucially important for the body to elicit a healthy response to an exercise stimulus. Another benefit of variable cyclic training is that it is much more interesting and has lower drop-out rates than long boring steady state cardio programs.

To summarize, some of the potential benefits of variable cyclic training compared to steady state endurance training are as follows: improved cardiovascular health, increased anti-oxidant protection, improved immune function, reduced risk for joint wear and tear, reduced muscle wasting, increased residual metabolic rate following exercise, and an increased capacity for the heart to handle life's every day stressors. There are many ways you can reap the benefits of stop-and-go or variable intensity physical training. One of the absolute most effective forms of variable intensity training to really reduce body fat and bring out serious muscular definition is performing wind sprints or hill sprints. Also, most competitive sports such as football, basketball, racquetball, tennis, hockey, etc. are naturally comprised of highly variable stop-and-go motion. In addition, weight training naturally incorporates short bursts of exertion followed by recovery periods. High intensity interval training (varying between high and low intensity intervals on any piece of cardio equipment) is yet another training method that utilizes exertion and recovery periods. For example, an interval training session on the treadmill could look something like this:

- Warm-up for 3-4 minutes at a fast walk or light jog
- Interval 1 - run at 8.0 mi/hr for 1 minute
- Interval 2 - walk at 4.0 mi/hr for 1.5 minutes
- Interval 3 - run at 10.0 mi/hr for 1 minute
- Interval 4 - walk at 4.0 mi/hr for 1.5 minutes

Repeat those 4 intervals 4 times for a very intense 20-minute workout.

The take-away message from this section is to try to train your body at highly variable intensity rates for the majority of your workouts to get the most beneficial response in terms of heart health, fat loss, and muscle maintenance.

2.2 Body Part Isolation vs. Complex Movements in Strength Training

Working as a fitness professional, there is one type of question I get all the time that shows that many people are missing the big picture regarding the benefits of strength training. This popular question usually goes something like this:

"What exercise can I do to isolate my _____ (insert your muscle of choice – abs, quads, biceps, triceps, etc)?"

It doesn't matter which muscle someone is asking about, they always seem to be asking how to 'isolate' it. My first response to this question is always – "Why in the world would you want to isolate it?"

The first thing I try to teach my clients is that the body does not work well in muscle isolation. Rather, it works better in movements along a kinetic chain; that is, large portions of the body assist other portions of the body in completing a complex movement. In fact, there really is no such thing as true muscle isolation. There is almost always a nearby muscle group that will assist in some way with whatever movement you are doing. However, this article compares attempting to 'isolate' body parts via single-joint exercises to the much more effective strategy of performing multi-joint complex movements.

When you attempt to 'isolate' muscles by performing single-joint exercises, you are actually creating a body that is non-functional and will be more prone to injury. Essentially, you are creating a body that is a compilation of body parts, instead of a powerful, functional unit that works together.

Now if you really want to end up hobbling around in a body bandaged up with joint problems, tendonitis, and excess body fat, then by all means, continue trying to 'isolate' body parts. On the other hand, if you would rather have a lean, muscular, injury-free, functional body that works as a complete powerful unit to perform complex movements (in athletics or even everyday tasks), then you need to shift your focus away from muscle isolation. Believe me, focusing on how well your body functions will give you the side effect of a body that looks even better than it would have if you focused on muscle isolation. For example, take a look at the physiques of any NFL running backs, wide receivers, or even world class sprinters. Trust me when I say that these guys pretty much NEVER train for muscle isolation (their strength coaches wouldn't be crazy enough to let them), yet they are absolutely ripped to shreds!

Another benefit to moving away from the 'muscle isolation' mindset to a more 'complex movement' mindset is that you will find it much easier to lose body fat. The reason is that by focusing more on multi-joint complex movements as opposed to single-joint muscle isolation, you not only burn a lot more calories during each workout, but you also increase your metabolic rate, and stimulate production of more fat burning and muscle building hormones like growth hormone and testosterone.

Let's look at an example. The machine leg extension is a single joint exercise that works mainly the quadriceps, can potentially cause knee joint instability in the long run, and doesn't even burn that many calories. On the other hand, exercises like squats, lunges, step-ups, and deadlifts are all multi-joint complex movements that work hundreds of muscles in the body (including the quadriceps) as a functional unit, create more stable and strong joints in the long run (when done properly), and also burn massive quantities of calories compared to the single-joint exercises.

2.3 Tired of the Same Old 3 Sets of 10? So is Your Body! Discover How to Manipulate Training Variables

Everyone will inadvertently hit a frustrating plateau in their training at one time or another. You're cruising along for a while, gaining strength, losing fat, looking better, and then all of the sudden it hits. Suddenly, you find yourself even weaker than before on your lifts, or you find that you've gained back a couple of pounds. It happens to everyone. Most of the time, these plateaus occur because people rarely change their training variables over time. Many people stick to the same types of exercises for the same basic sets and reps and rest periods with the same boring cardio routine. Well, I hope to open your mind and bring some creativity to your workouts with this section!

There are many ways that you can strategically modify your training variables to assure that you maximize your fat loss and/or muscle building response to exercise. Most people only think about changing their sets and reps performed, if they even think about changing their routine at all. However, other variables that can dramatically affect your results are changing the order of exercises (sequence), exercise grouping (super-setting, circuit training, tri-sets, etc.), exercise type (multi-joint or single joint, free-weight or machine based), the number of exercises per workout, the amount of resistance, the time under tension, the base of stability (standing, seated, on stability ball, one-legged, etc.), the volume of work (sets x reps x distance moved), rest periods between sets, repetition speed, range of motion, exercise angle (inclined, flat, declined, bent over, upright, etc), training duration per workout, and training frequency per week. Sounds like a lot of different training aspects to consider in order to achieve the best results from your workouts, doesn't it? Well, that's where a knowledgeable personal trainer can make sense of all of this for you to make sure that your training doesn't get stale. Below are a few examples to get your mind working to come up with more creative and result producing workouts.

Most people stick to workouts where they do something along the lines of 3 sets of 10-12 reps per exercise, with 2-3 minutes rest between sets. Booooorrrrring!!!! Here are a few examples of different methods to spice up your routine.

- Try 10 sets of 3, with only 20 seconds rest between sets.
- Try using a fairly heavy weight and complete 6 sets of 6 reps, doing a 3 minute treadmill sprint between each weight lifting set.
- Try using a near maximum weight and do 10 sets of 1 rep, with only 30 seconds rest between sets.
- Try using a lighter than normal weight and do 1 set of 50 reps for each exercise
- Try a workout based on only one full body exercise, such as barbell clean & presses or dumbbell squat & presses, and do nothing but that exercise for an intense 20 minutes.
- Try a workout based on all bodyweight exercises such as pushups, pull-ups, chin-ups, dips, bodyweight squats, lunges, up and down stairs, etc.
- Try a circuit of 12 different exercises covering the entire body without any rest between exercises.
- Try that same 12 exercise circuit on your subsequent workout, but do the entire circuit in the reverse order.
- Try your usual exercises at a faster repetition speed on one workout and then at a super-slow speed on your next workout.
- Try completing six 30 minute workouts one week, followed by three 1-hr workouts the next week. This will keep your body guessing.
- Try doing drop sets of all of your exercises, where you drop the weight between each set and keep doing repetitions without any rest until complete muscular fatigue (usually about 5-6 sets in a row).

There are many more ways to continue to change your training variables. This was just a taste of your possibilities. Be creative and get results!

2.4 Your Workouts Need Both Consistency and Variability for Max Results

In the last chapter, I spoke about the fact that you must alter your training variables that make up your workouts if you want to continuously get good results, whether it is losing weight, building muscle, or toning up.

While changing your training variables is an integral part of the success of your training program, your workouts shouldn't be drastically different every single time. If you are all over the place on each workout and never try to repeat and improve on specific exercises for specific set and rep schemes with specific rest intervals, then your body has no basis to improve on its current condition. The best way to structure your workouts to get the best results is to be consistent and try to continually improve on a specific training method for a specific time period. A time period of 4-8 weeks usually works best as your body will adapt to the specific training method and progress will slow after this amount of time.

At this point, it is time to change around some of your training variables as I described in the "exercise variables" article, and then stay consistent with your new training program for another 4-8 weeks. To refresh, some of these variables are the numbers of sets and reps of exercises, the order of exercises (sequence), exercise grouping (super-setting, circuit training, tri-sets, etc.), exercise type (multi-joint or single joint, free-weight or machine based), the number of exercises per workout, the amount of resistance, the time under tension, the base of stability (standing, seated, on stability ball, one-legged, etc.), the volume of work (sets x reps x distance moved), rest periods between sets, repetition speed, range of motion, exercise angle (inclined, flat, declined, bent over, upright, etc), training duration per workout, training frequency per week, etc.

For example, let's say you are training with a program where you are doing 10 sets of 3 reps for 6 different exercises grouped together in pairs (done as supersets) with 30 seconds rest between each superset and no rest between the 2 exercises within the superset. If you are smart, I'm sure you are tracking your progress with a notepad (weights used, sets, and reps) to see how you are progressing over time. Let's say that after about 6 weeks, you find that you are no longer improving with that program. Well, now it is time to change up your variables, and start a new program.

This time you might choose a classic 5 sets of 5 reps routine, but you group your exercises in tri-sets (three exercises performed back to back to back, and then repeated for the number of sets). This time you decide to perform the exercises in the tri-set with no rest between them, and then recover for 2 minutes in between each tri-set to fully recoup your strength levels.

2.5 The Ultimate Hard-Body Exercise

As you may have already discovered, the squat is at the top of the heap (along with deadlifts) as one of the most effective overall exercises for stimulating body composition changes (muscle gain and fat loss). This is because exercises like squats and deadlifts use more muscle groups under a heavy load than almost any other weight bearing exercises known to man. Hence, these exercises stimulate the greatest hormonal responses (growth hormone, testosterone, etc.) of all exercises. In fact, university research studies have even proven that inclusion of squats into a training program increases upper body development, in addition to lower body development, even though upper body specific joint movements are not performed during the squat. Whether your goal is gaining muscle mass, losing body fat, building a strong and functional body, or improving athletic performance, the basic squat and deadlift (and their variations) are the ultimate solution. If you don't believe me that squats and deadlifts are THE basis for a lean and powerful body, then go ahead and join all of the other overweight people pumping away mindlessly for hours on boring cardio equipment. You won't find long boring cardio in any of my programs!

Squats can be done simply with your bodyweight or with any free weighted objects for extra resistance such as barbells, dumbbells, kettlebells, sandbags, etc. Squats should only be done with free weights – NEVER with a Smith machine or any other squat machines! Machines do not allow your body to follow natural, biomechanically-correct movement paths. You also perform less work because the machine stabilizes the weight for you. Therefore, you get weaker results!

The type of squat that people are most familiar with is the barbell back squat where the bar is resting on the trapezius muscles of the upper back. Many professional strength coaches believe that front squats (where the bar rests on the shoulders in front of the head) and overhead squats (where the bar is locked out in a snatch grip overhead throughout the squat) are more functional to athletic performance than back squats with less risk of lower back injury. I feel that a combination of all three (not necessarily during the same phase of your workouts) will yield the best results for overall muscular development, body fat loss, and athletic performance. Front squats are moderately more difficult than back squats, while overhead squats are considerably more difficult than either back squats or front squats. I'll cover overhead squats in a future article. If you are only accustomed to performing back squats, it will take you a few sessions to become comfortable with front squats, so start out light. After a couple sessions of practice, you will start to feel the groove and be able to increase the poundage. Let's take a closer look at front squats in particular.

To perform front squats:

The front squat recruits the abdominals to a much higher degree for stability due to the more upright position compared with back squats. It is mostly a lower body exercise, but is great for functionally incorporating core strength and stability into the squatting movement. It can also be slightly difficult to learn how to properly rest the bar on your shoulders. There are two ways to rest the bar on the front of the shoulders. In the first method, you step under the bar and cross your forearms into an "X" position while resting the bar on the dimple that is created by the shoulder muscle near the bone, keeping your elbows up high so that your arms are parallel to the ground. You then hold the bar in place by pressing the thumb side of your fists against the bar for support. Alternatively, you can hold the bar by placing your palms face up and the bar resting on your fingers against your shoulders. For both methods, your elbows must stay up high to prevent the weight from falling. Your upper arms should stay parallel to the ground throughout the squat. Find out which bar support method is more comfortable for you. Then, initiate the squat from your hips by sitting back and down, keeping the weight on your heels as opposed to the balls of your feet. Squat down to a position where your thighs are approximately parallel to the ground, then press back up to the starting position. Keeping your weight more towards your heels is the key factor in squatting to protect your knees from injury and develop strong injury-resistant knee joints. Keep in mind – squats done correctly actually strengthen the knees; squats done incorrectly can damage the knees. Practice first with an un-weighted bar or a relatively light weight to learn the movement. Most people are surprised how hard this exercise works your abs once you learn the correct form. This is due to the more upright posture compared with back squats.

2.6 Barbell, Kettlebell, and Dumbbell Complexes - a Different Style of Weight Training for a Ripped Body

If you've been looking for a different training technique to break out of a rut, eliminate the boredom, and bring on new results, "complexes" may be just what you've been looking for. If you've never heard of "complexes" before, the basic concept is that instead of repeating the same exercise for multiple reps to complete a "set", you sequence one rep of several different exercises right after one another and repeat the sequence several times to complete a "set". No, this is NOT circuit training...it's much different. It's basically like performing a routine, instead of just mindlessly performing a typical "set". This type of training is excellent to work a huge amount of musculature in a short amount of time, and definitely takes your workouts to a whole new level of intensity. The conditioning aspect of this type of training is amazing, as you'll find yourself huffing and puffing after repeating a sequence a mere two or three times. If I had to venture a guess, I'd have to say that this type of training probably elicits a good growth hormone response as well, due to the large amount of full body work completed in a given time period. But that's just my guess.

I like to incorporate about 5 exercises into my complexes. Any more than that and you might start to forget what's next in the sequence. Here's an example of a killer barbell complex that really gets me fired up:

Example Barbell Complex

1. high pull from floor (explosive deadlift right into upright row in one motion);

2. barbell back to thighs, then hang clean (explosively pull bar from knees and "catch" the bar at shoulders);

3. barbell back to floor, then clean & push-press;

4. barbell back to thighs, bend over, then bent over row;

5. barbell back to thighs, then finish with Romanian deadlift

Use a weight that you can still handle for your weakest lift of the bunch, but keep it heavy enough to challenge you. Try to repeat the sequence 2-3 times without resting... That's 1 set. You could progress over time on this routine by increasing the amount of times you repeat the sequence in each set, or by adding sets on subsequent workouts before eventually increasing the weight. For example, say you completed the above complex with 155-lbs for 3 sequences per set for 3 sets in today's workout. Next time you perform the workout, try to do 155 lbs for 3 sequences per set for 4 sets. Once you successfully complete 5 sets with 155, increase the weight 5 or 10 lbs next time, and drop back to 3 sets. This is a great way to make improvements over time, while cycling your training volume.

Now I'm going to show you a great kettlebell complex that really kicks my butt. I've been training with kettlebells for a little over a year now, and can definitely say that they've dramatically improved my strength, body composition, and overall physical capabilities. If you're not familiar with kettlebells, they are an old eastern European training secret that has just started to take the US by storm over the last few years. Many elite athletes are using kettlebells as their preferred training tool for serious results. You can learn more info about body-hardening [kettlebells here](). I'd recommend just starting off with one bell and learn all of the single kettlebell drills first, before delving into the double-bell drills. Just one kettlebell coupled with some bodyweight exercises can literally be enough to comprise your own home gym, without any other equipment necessary. Or you can just incorporate kettlebell training into your normal training routine once or twice a week to shake up your routine and stimulate new results. Either way, they are one of the best fitness products I've ever invested in that I'll be able to use for the rest of my life.

Example Kettlebell Complex

1. one arm swing

2. one arm snatch, keep the bell over head;

3. one arm overhead squat;

4. bell back down to bottom, then one arm split snatch;

5. bell back down to bottom, then one arm clean & press

As with the barbell complex, repeat the sequence (without rest) 2-3 times with each arm. That's one set...and one hell of a killer set at that! Try increasing from 3 to 4 to 5 sets on subsequent workouts with a given weight before increasing your sequence reps. If you're not drenched in sweat with your heart beating out of your chest after that complex, you either went too light, or you are a mutant freak!

Alright, since most people will have easier access to dumbbells instead of kettlebells, now I'll show you how to compile a good dumbbell complex.

Example Dumbbell Complex

1. upright row with each arm separately, then both together;

2. front lunge with one leg, then the other;

3. back lunge with one leg, then the other;

4. curl to overhead press;

5. keep dumbbells at shoulders and squat

Again, the same type of sequencing and progressions work great with the dumbbell complexes. I think a great strategy is to alternate barbell complexes on one day with kettlebell or dumbbell complexes on alternative training days. For example, you could do barbell complexes Monday, K-bell or D-bell complexes Wednesday, and back to barbell complexes on Friday. Maybe hit some sprints and bodyweight drills on Saturday or Sunday; then Monday would be K-bell or D-bell complexes again, Wednesday would be barbells again, and so on. Give this program a try for a month (if you dare), and you will be one hardened individual!

2.7 Top 15 Non-Traditional, Muscle-Building, Fat Blasting Workouts!

If you have been a subscriber to my newsletter for some time, you know that I'm always trying to give you ways to make your workouts more interesting and fun, while also stimulating big-time results. Don't you agree that your training should be fun? This is what separates the people who jump on and off the "fitness bandwagon" a couple times every year without ever making any real progress from the people that actually adopt a true fitness lifestyle and finally achieve the body they have always wanted. Make it interesting, make it fun, and make your fitness a priority, and you'll have the body that you want.

What I have noticed over the years is that many people will train regularly for a few months and then will either get bored with the same old weight training and cardio routines, or will get discouraged because their progress comes to a grinding halt after a while. In my opinion, I don't think your workouts ever need to get boring or stale. You just need to have an open mind to the huge world of various training styles and techniques that are out there. Seriously, there are so many different and fun training styles out there, that there is no reason you should ever get bored with your workouts and give up on that lean ripped body that you've been looking for. Also, mixing in various training styles builds stronger joints by reducing repetitive movement pattern overload and varying your training stressors.

Now before I start with some of my favorite non-traditional training styles, I will state that I think one of the best ways to achieve a lean, muscular and healthy body is through a consistent weight training routine with free weights. You can choose to integrate some of these alternative training techniques with your weight training routines on the same day, as alternative workouts on separate days of the week, or even as separate training cycles where you try some of these techniques for several weeks at a time before cycling back to a traditional weight training workout. Try some of these training styles out and you'll be on your way to never being bored again with your workouts…and your body will thank you with muscles popping out that you never knew existed!

Alright, here are some of my favorite non-traditional training techniques:

1. Staircase Workouts – This is great because stairs are everywhere. You can go to a football field and do stadium stairs, any building that has stairs like a hotel (most people take the elevator, so you won't even have many people looking at you while you're working out), or even the stairs in your own home. For an awesome full body workout, try mixing stairs sprints with an upper body exercise like pushups or pull-ups. If done with a high enough intensity, stairs workouts help to create changes throughout your entire body due to the muscle building and fat burning hormonal response and metabolism increase that you get through working the biggest muscle groups in your entire body. If you thought that going up and down the stairs was the only way to get a good stairs workout…think again.

2. Wind Sprints and Hill Sprints – Find any open field in a park or athletic field and try 50, 75, and 100-yard all-out wind sprints. After each sprint, rest long enough to catch your breath before the next one (generally 1-2 minutes). Try workouts of anywhere from 6 to 20 wind sprints for a great "cutting" workout. Also, if you have a hill nearby, hill sprints are also great workouts. Sprint up the hill as fast as you can and walk down for your rest interval. Repeat until you're whooped. These sprint workouts are so amazingly effective at changing your entire body for the same reason as stairs exercises…by powerfully working the biggest muscle groups in your entire body, you greatly stimulate your metabolism while simultaneously increasing your fat burning and muscle building hormones. Just look at any world class 100-meter sprinters and notice how ripped-to-shreds those guys

are. Now compare that to the emaciated weakling physiques of many marathoners, and you'll see that sprinting is where the action is at for a healthy, ripped, powerful body! Now I don't want to upset all of you distance runners out there. Hey, if distance running is something you enjoy, then go right ahead. But don't say you're doing it for the health benefits, because I might just have to disagree. Section 2.1 in this book provided my full opinion on why I believe highly variable intensity exercise (such as sprinting and interval training) is far superior to steady state endurance exercise (such as jogging, endurance cycling, or any same-pace cardio).

3. Kettlebell Training – You've probably heard me praise kettlebell training many times before, but I will have to reiterate that it has been one of the best training methods that I've ever tried and has taken my physical capabilities to a whole new level. Kettlebells are an alternative type of free-weight training instead of barbells and dumbbells. Their unique construction and weight distribution (basically a cannonball with a handle) allows for a whole different realm of exercises that's available compared to dumbbells and barbells. Kettlebells have been typically used for training hard-core athletes, military units, martial arts competitors, and other tough individuals, but there is no reason that anybody looking to get stronger, bigger, or more cut can't learn the exercises and benefit from them. It's been a little over a year now since I've incorporated kettlebell training into my routines, and I'll admit that I'm hooked for life! At between $100-$150 per kettlebell, they are definitely not cheap, but they are well worth the money. Just one or two kettlebells and you've literally got yourself an entire home gym that you can use for the rest of your life…worth every penny in my book!

4. Bodyweight Workouts – Try doing one or two workouts a week at home with just bodyweight based exercises. These can be great because you can get a high intensity workout done in only 15-30 minutes without having to go to the gym on days that you might not have time for a trip to the gym. Try

alternating bodyweight squats, pushups variations, lunges, and floor abs exercises continuously for 15-30 minutes. Try to take very short rest periods or none at all to really amp up the intensity since this will be a brief workout. If you're more advanced, you can even incorporate more challenging exercises like handstand pushups, one-arm pushups, and one-legged squats into your bodyweight training routines. For those of you that want to develop crushing strength through bodyweight exercises alone, a great book that I read a couple years back is called the Naked Warrior by Pavel Tsatsouline.

5. Ring Training – This type of training basically uses portable gymnastic rings that you can take anywhere with you. You throw the straps up over any high bar like a pullup bar, the top of a power rack, or even over a football field goal crossbar. Then you can quickly adjust the rings to do exercises like ring dips, ring pushups, ring pull-ups, hanging leg raises, horizontal body rows, L-sits, and more. Dips and pushups on the rings are my favorites and the rings really make them a hell of a lot more difficult, while also incorporating your stabilizer muscles to a much greater degree. The rings allow your joints to move in a more natural pattern and can help you prevent or even recover from shoulder injuries. Personally, when I try dips on a normal dip stand, it hurts my shoulders. However, dips on the training rings feel perfect, and also give me a much better muscle pump. The training rings are one of the best training devices I've ever bought. Give them a try…I think you'll like them if you're up for a challenge. Ever notice the impressive upper body development of gymnasts… yep, that's mostly due to the rings!

6. Swimming – A great full body workout that stresses the muscles and joints in a much different way than most resistance training. Incorporating swimming workouts once or twice a week into your normal training routings can really enhance your physique. I recommend trying a "sprint" style swimming workout, which will help more for building muscle compared with

endurance long distance swimming. For sprint style, swim as hard as you can to the other side of a 25-meter or 50-meter pool (or sprint swim similar distances in a lake or the ocean if you like to swim outdoors). Rest enough to catch your breath between sprint swims (about 20-40 seconds). Try to keep the rest intervals fairly short with swim sprints. You can also mix different strokes (crawl, breaststroke, sidestroke, backstroke, butterfly) on each swim sprint. I've found that sprint swimming gives me a great muscle pump (especially in the upper body), without any soreness the next day as is typical with weight training. This is because swimming has no eccentric movement (the negative portion of a lift), which is what causes muscle soreness. You can get a great sprint swimming workout done in about 30-40 minutes. Keep in mind that even though swimming works your muscles well and is a great alternative workout to mix in once or twice a week, it does not strengthen your bones. You still need to do regular weight training to do that.

7. Sandbag Training – This form of training is a nice variation to mix in with your strength training. It works your body with an unstable object, which makes muscles that might normally be neglected get in on the action to perform the movements. I've been mixing some sandbag training into my routines for over a year now, and I've found it is a very intense method of training that works your muscles in a different way and gets you huffing and puffing like crazy. You can make your own sandbags to train with by filling various sized duffle bags with sand, or you can use those construction type sandbags that come in several shapes. Sandbag exercises can be done as squats, cleans, presses, lunges, shouldering, throws or heaves, carrying up hills, etc. Make no mistake…adding intense sandbag training to your routine will have you ripped in no time! I've actually read an entire book recently devoted to sandbag training, which gave me some really good ideas for sandbag based workouts.

8. Mountain Biking – As you may have figured out by now, I'm not a proponent of steady pace endurance exercise, but rather, highly variable intensity exercise that works with bursts of exertion followed by recovery intervals. Well, mountain biking fits this bill perfectly. You get the leg pumping exertion during the uphill climbs, while also getting the adrenaline rush of the downhill acting as your recovery intervals. Mix it all together and you get a super-fun, high-intensity, leg burning workout that will melt fat off of your entire body and build awesome legs at the same time. The climbs can be tough and will challenge you both physically and mentally as you pump away trying to make it up steep hills without having to resort to getting off of the bike. Then after you make it up the challenging climbs, you get rewarded with the adrenaline rush of flying down steep hills while jumping off of boulders and logs and trying not to stumble or fall off the bike. It's such an addicting thrill…I love it! See, who says that working out has to be boring!

9. Indoor (or outdoor) Rock Climbing – This is yet another fun way to get in a great workout that will also challenge you both physically and mentally. Indoor rock climbing gyms have starting popping up all over the place in recent years and will be more accessible than outdoor rock climbing to most people. Rock climbing is a great workout for your legs, arms, shoulders, and your entire back. It also really works your grip strength and forearms like crazy. Whenever I go indoor rock climbing (which is only on occasion), my forearms are sore for about 2-3 days afterwards. Give it a try if you've never done it…it may be just what you're looking for to spice up your fitness routine.

10. Stick Wrestling – This is a killer full body workout and can also be a great competition between you and your friends. This is probably more of a guy thing for most. You could even come up with your own "fight club" and have stick wrestling competitions with your buddies to see who is toughest. There are actually sticks designed specifically for stick wresting, but you can even

just use a strong broomstick cut down to about 30-36 inches long and taped up with some athletic tape to prevent splinters. For your stick wrestling workout, stand on a soft mat or carpeted area (or grass if outdoors), match up with a friend or foe. You'll both grab the same stick toward the ends with your hands on the outsides of your partner's hands, on the inside, or staggered. Then you simply push, pull, jerk, and thrash your opponent around trying to knock them off balance until they either fall or lose their grip of the stick…and you win that round! Be careful not to get the stick up high and knock each other in the face. Use common sense. You can do this in 1-2 minute rounds or just keep going until someone gives up. Be creative and keep going until you've gotten a killer workout. Your forearms and legs will be screaming!

11. Strongman Training – This type of training is a little more hard-core, but it's a blast for those who are into trying something different. The premise is based on the types of exercises competitors perform in the "worlds strongest man" competitions. If you have a yard, you can even set up some of these exercises in your yard and do some outdoor workouts to have a little fun. You can get one of those giant tractor tires and do tire flips (which is basically a deadlift followed by a push-press). You can also try your hand at log lifts, boulder lifts and carries, keg lifts and tosses, sled dragging…anything that involves pulling, pushing, lifting, or heaving any types of odd objects. You don't need to be a monster to enjoy this type of training…just handle whatever size objects are challenging for your individual strength. Strongman training works your entire body in a very intense fashion and could easily spark some new results.

12. Rope Climbing – This goes back to the old high school days of climbing the rope in gym class. Seriously, if you have access to a rope, either at a gym or somewhere outdoors, rope climbing builds a powerful and ripped upper

body like no other exercise. A great way to incorporate rope climbing into intense workouts is to do a climb up, then lower yourself back down. Then while your upper body is recovering for the next climb, you can do a lower body exercise like squats or lunges, or go up and down stairs. Keep alternating the upper body rope climbs with the lower body exercises in between and you'll get one hell of a full body workout.

13. Bag Boxing – You can use a heavy bag, a speed bag, or even one of those rebound bags to get a great workout. Among the three, the heavy bag is the best all around full body workout, while the speed bag will test your rhythm and timing and give you a great upper body workout. If available at your gym or if you have a bag at home, try mixing these in as a good warm-up or as an intense finish to your strength routine.

14. Rope Skipping – You can't beat rope jumping as a great full body exercise. I like to use it as a warm-up for my weight training workouts. I prefer to use the really cheap "speed" ropes with a plastic rope instead of a fabric rope. Once you get good, you can jump rope much faster with the plastic ropes than the fabric ones, which will allow you to get a more intense workout. Try mixing together two legged jumps, one-legged jumps, arm crossovers, double jumps (rope passes under feet twice for each jump) to keep things interesting and increase the intensity. Also, try alternating 15-20 second high intensity bursts where you jump as fast as you possibly can, followed by 15-20 second recovery intervals where you jump slowly to get ready for your next burst. Keep repeating until you're whooped.

15. Jumping exercises – squat jumps, box jumps, lunge jumps, and broad jumps are some of the best ways to incorporate explosive jumping exercises into your routines. The explosive and powerful nature of jumping exercises works your leg muscles in an entirely different way than most normal slow grinding strength training moves. I've even seen a university study cited once that found squat jumps to elicit the greatest testosterone response of

Well, I hope you've enjoyed all of these ideas for ways to really shake up your workouts and make them fun again. I know some of them may seem a little "out there", but open your mind to the possibilities and you'll never be bored again…and your body will respond with new found results! Remember, don't listen to all of the gimmicks and infomercials, etc. that claim that THEIR training style or machine or routine is THE BEST in the world. There is no single "best" method. But there are lots of great methods to try out and see which work best for you and keeps you interested!

Nutrition is next…

3.0 NUTRITION STRATEGIES

3.1 Post-Workout Nutrition: Secrets to a Hard, Lean Body

As you've probably heard before, your post-workout meal may very well be your most important meal of the day. The reason is that when you're finished with an intense workout, you're entering a catabolic state where your muscle glycogen is depleted and increased cortisol levels are beginning to excessively break down muscle tissue. These conditions (if left to go too long) are not good and the only way to reverse this catabolic state (and promote an anabolic state) is to consume a quickly digestible post-workout meal as soon as you can after training. The goal is to choose a meal with quickly digestible carbs to replenish muscle glycogen as well as quickly digestible protein to provide the amino acids needed to jump start muscular repair. The surge of carbohydrates and amino acids from this quickly digested meal promotes an insulin spike from the pancreas, which shuttles nutrients into the muscle cells. The post-workout meal should generally contain between 300-500 calories to get the best response. For example, a 120-lb female may only need a 300-calorie meal, whereas a 200-lb male may need a 500-calorie post-workout meal. Your post-workout meal should also contain anywhere from a 2:1 ratio of carbs:protein to a 4:1 ratio of carbs:protein. While most of your other daily meals should contain a source of healthy fats, keep the fat content of your post-workout meal to a bare minimum, since fat slows the absorption of the meal, which is the opposite of what you want after a workout.

When choosing what to make for your post-workout meal, the first thing to realize is that you DON'T need any of these expensive post-workout supplement formulations that the magazines (who advertise for them) will tell you that you absolutely NEED! As with any nutritional strategies, natural is always better. A good source of quickly digestible natural carbs such as frozen bananas, pineapples, raisins, honey, or organic maple syrup are perfect to elicit an insulin response that will promote muscle glycogen replenishment and a general anabolic (muscle building) effect. The best source of quickly digestible protein is a quality non-denatured whey protein isolate, some fat-free or low-fat yogurt, or even some fat free or low fat ricotta cheese. Ricotta is mostly whey protein, so it is fast digesting. Cottage cheese, on the other hand, is mostly casein and is slow digesting and would not be good as a post-workout meal (even though it is great any other time of day). Here are a couple ideas for delicious post-workout smoothies that will kick start your recovery process:

Chocolate Banana – blend together 1 cup water, ½ cup skim milk, one and a half frozen bananas, 2 tbsp organic maple syrup, and 30 grams chocolate whey protein powder – 38 g prot, 72 g carb, 0.5 g fat, 440 calories.

Pineapple Vanilla - blend together 1 cup water, ½ cup vanilla yogurt, one cup frozen pineapples, 2 tbsp honey (preferably raw), and 30 grams vanilla whey protein powder – 35 g prot, 71 g carb, 0.5 g fat, 425 calories.

When looking to lose body fat, keep in mind that post-workout meals should have the opposite characteristics of all of your other meals throughout each day. While post-workout meals should have quick high glycemic index carbs, quickly digested proteins, and minimal fat, all of your other meals throughout the day should be comprised of low glycemic index, slowly digested carbs, slow release proteins, and ample healthy fats. These are powerful strategies towards developing a lean muscular body with a low body fat percentage. Another great thing about post-workout meals is that you can satisfy even the worst sweet tooth, since this is the one time of the day where you can get away with eating extra sugars without adding to your gut. Instead, it all goes straight to the muscles! Enjoy!

3.2 Don't be Afraid of Dietary Fat! Even Some Saturated Fats are Healthy for You

I'll preface this section by saying that it will help if you have an open mind and accept that some of these facts are a slap in the face to politically correct nutrition in this day and age where fats are admonished by many well intentioned, but mislead health professionals, doctors, the mass media, etc.

To start, eating an adequate supply of healthy dietary fats is vitally important to your overall health. Fats are one of the main components in all of the cell membranes throughout your entire body. If you eat enough healthy natural fats, your cellular processes will proceed normally. On the other hand, if you eat man-made, heavily processed, chemically altered fats (damaged fats) that are found in most processed foods, your cellular function will be impaired as these damaged fats become part of your cell membranes, the body will have to work harder to operate correctly, and degenerative diseases can develop. In addition, healthy dietary fats are essential for optimal hormone production and balance within the body and are therefore essential for the muscle building and fat burning processes. Did you know that eating a diet that is too low in fat will reduce your testosterone levels? You know what the results of that are: less muscle and more fat on your frame. Females, don't be afraid…your testosterone is not going to go through the roof by eating more fat. It helps to keep everything in balance for both men and women, as long as you eat the right fats (more on the right fats in a minute). Other important functions that dietary fats play in a healthy body are aiding vitamin and mineral utilization, enzyme regulation, energy, etc.

I cringe every time I hear so called "health experts" recommend restriction of dietary fat, claiming that a low-fat diet is the key to good health, weight loss, and prevention of degenerative diseases. Restriction of any one macronutrient (protein, carbs, or fat) in your diet works against what your body needs and can only lead to problems. All three basic macronutrients serve important functions for a lean, healthy, and disease-free body. As Dr. Mary Enig, Ph.D, and one of the leading fats and lipids researchers in the world notes in several of her books and articles, there is very little true scientific evidence supporting the assertion that a high fat diet is bad for us. For example, if these so called "health experts" that admonish fat are correct, and a low-fat diet is the solution to good health, then why did traditional Pacific Islanders who typically obtained 2/3 to 3/4 of their total daily calories from fat (mostly from coconut fat), remain virtually free from heart disease, obesity, and other modern degenerative diseases (that is, until Western dietary influences invaded)? Also, why did traditional Eskimo populations, consuming up to 75% of their total caloric intake from fat (mostly from whale blubber, seal fat, organ meats, and cold water fish), display superior health and longevity without heart disease or obesity? Why did members of the Masai tribe in Africa remain free from degenerative diseases and maintain low body fat percentages on diets consisting of large quantities of raw whole milk, blood, and meat? What about the Samburu tribe of Africa, which eats an average of 5 times the quantity of dietary fat (mostly from raw whole milk and meat) as overweight, disease-ridden Americans, yet Samburu members are lean, healthy, and free of degenerative diseases? What about traditional Mediterranean diets, which are known to be very high in fat (sometimes up to 70% fat), and are also well known to be very healthy?

These examples of high fat diets and the associated excellent health of traditional populations around the world go on and on, yet it seems that many doctors, nutritionists, and government agencies still ignore these facts and continue to promote a diet that restricts fat intake. It's not that their intentions are bad, it's just that everyone has been brainwashed by poor science over the years, when in fact, there really is no hard evidence that **natural unprocessed** fats are bad for us.

Well, the problem that has led to this misconception is that the good fats (the natural, unprocessed, health promoting fats) have gotten mistakenly lumped together in nutritional advice with the deadly processed fats and oils that make up a large percentage of almost all processed food that is sold at your local grocery store, restaurant, deli, fast food joint, etc. These deadly processed fats are literally everywhere and almost impossible to avoid unless you know what to look for and make smart choices in what you feed your body with. Take note that I'm not recommending following a super high fat diet. Active individuals that exercise on a regular basis certainly also need adequate supplies of healthy carbohydrates for energy and muscle glycogen replenishment, as well as good sources of protein for muscle repair. The above examples of the high fat diets of traditional populations and their corresponding excellent health were simply to prove the point that you don't need to be afraid of dietary fats as long as you make healthy natural choices and stay within your daily caloric range to maintain or lose weight (depending on your goals). Following is a list of some of the healthiest fatty foods (some will surprise you!) as well as some of the deadliest fatty foods to try to avoid at all costs:

The Healthy Fatty Food Choices:
- Coconut fat (and other tropical oils): Coconut fat is approximately 92% saturated fat, yet surprisingly to most people, is considered a very healthy natural fat. The health benefits of coconut fat lie in its composition of approximately 65% medium chain triglycerides (MCTs). Specifically, about 50% of coconut fat is a MCT called lauric acid, which has very potent anti-microbial properties helping to enhance the immune system. Also, MCTs are more easily utilized for immediate energy instead of being stored as body fat. Coconut oil is also an excellent cooking oil for stir-frying, baking, etc. since saturated fats are much more stable and do not oxidize like polyunsaturated oils when exposed to heat and light, which creates damaging free radicals. The best sources of healthy coconut fat are organic coconut milk, virgin coconut oil, or fresh coconut. Palm oil (non-hydrogenated) is another healthy tropical oil that is highly saturated. Keep in mind that most mainstream health and fitness professionals have been brainwashed to believe that tropical oils are unhealthy. So you will see other health professionals all over the place writing statements such as "avoid saturated fats at all costs" and similar. Come on now. Think about it. A large portion of our natural food supply on this planet is composed of saturated fats, substances that we humans are meant to eat and thrive on. It is only

when we humans take natural food and put it through all kinds of chemical and physical processing (that it was never meant to undergo naturally), that it becomes unhealthy.

- Extra virgin olive oil: Olive oil is approximately 71% monounsaturated, 16% saturated, and 13% polyunsaturated. Choose "extra virgin" olive oil, which comes from the first pressing of the olives and has higher quantities of antioxidants. Unlike most other oils on supermarket shelves, extra virgin olive oil is not extracted with the use of harmful industrial solvents and is one of your healthiest choices for liquid oils. Try making your own salad dressing by mixing a small amount of olive oil with vinegar. This is healthier than most store bought salad dressings, which are usually made with highly processed and refined (chemically damaged) soybean oil extracted with industrial solvents.
- Dark, bittersweet chocolate (>70% cocoa content): The cocoa bean is a very concentrated source of antioxidants and responsible for part of the health benefit of dark chocolate. The fat portion of the cocoa bean (cocoa butter) is a healthy natural fat, composed of approximately 59% saturated fat (mostly healthy stearic acid), 38% monounsaturated fat, and 3% polyunsaturated fat. I'll limit the description of healthy chocolate to ONLY dark bittersweet chocolate with >70% cocoa content. Most milk chocolates are only about 30% cocoa, and even most dark chocolates are only about 50% cocoa, leaving the remainder of those products composed of high amounts of sugar, milk fat, corn sweeteners, etc. Look for a quality dark chocolate that lists its cocoa content between 70%-80%. A dark chocolate with cocoa content in this range will contain mostly cocoa and very little sugar, but still have a mildly sweet taste with a smooth and creamy texture. Keep in mind that although dark chocolate can be a healthy treat, it is still calorie dense, so keeping it to just a square or two is a good idea.

- Avocados or guacamole: The fat in avocados (depending on where they're grown) is approximately 60% monounsaturated, 25% saturated, and 15% polyunsaturated. Avocados are a very healthy natural food that provides many nutrients, fiber, and healthful fats, while adding a rich flavor to any meal. Try sliced avocado on sandwiches or in salads or use guacamole in wraps, sandwiches, or quesadillas.
- High fat fish such as wild salmon, sardines, mackerel, herring, trout, etc.: Just about any fish or seafood are good sources of natural omega-3 polyunsaturated fats, but the higher fat fish listed above are the best sources of omega-3's. Due to the radical switch to a higher proportion of omega-6 polyunsaturated fats like soybean oil, corn oil, safflower oil, etc. in our food supply during the middle of the 20th century, the average western diet is currently way too high in omega-6's compared to omega-3's, which wreaks havoc in your body. This is where good omega-3 sources like high fat fish, walnuts, and flax seeds can help bring you back to a better ratio of omega-6/omega-3.
- Nuts (any and all - walnuts, almonds, peanuts, cashews, macadamias, etc.): Nuts are great sources of healthy unprocessed fats as well as minerals and other trace nutrients. Macadamias, almonds, and cashews are great sources of monounsaturated fats, while walnuts are a good source of unprocessed polyunsaturated fats (including omega-3's). Try to avoid nuts that are cooked in oil. Instead, choose raw or dry roasted nuts.
- Seeds (sunflower seeds, pumpkin seeds, sesame seeds, flax seeds, etc.): All of these seeds are great sources of natural unprocessed healthy fats. In particular, flax seeds have received a lot of attention lately due to their high omega-3 content. However, keep in mind that omega-3 polyunsaturated fats are highly reactive to heat and light, and prone to oxidation and free radical production, so freshly ground flax seed is the only way to go. Instead of using the store bought ground flax seed, you can buy whole flax seed and use one of those miniature coffee grinders to grind your own flax seed. Try grinding fresh flax seed into your yogurt, cereal, or even your salad. If you're using flax oil, make sure it's a cold-pressed oil in a light-proof

refrigerated container, and use it up within a few weeks to prevent it from going rancid. NEVER cook with flax oil!

- The fat in organically raised, free-range animals: This is one area where most people have been misinformed by the mass media. Animal fat is inherently good for us, that is, if it came from a **healthy animal**. Human beings have thrived on animal fats for thousands of years. The problem lies in the fact that most mass produced animal products today do NOT come from healthy animals. They come from animals given loads of antibiotics and fattened up with hormones and fed un-natural feed. The solution is to choose organically raised, free-range meats, eggs, and dairy. At this time, the price is still a little higher, but it is worth it, and as demand grows, the prices will come down.

The Deadly Fatty Foods:

- Hydrogenated oils (source of artificial trans fats): These are industrially produced chemically altered oils subjected to extremely high pressure and temperature, with added industrial solvents such as hexane for extraction, and have a metal catalyst added to promote the artificial hydrogenation, followed by bleaching and deodorizing agents…..and somehow the FDA still allows this crap to pass as food. These oils aren't even worthy of your lawnmower, much less your body! They've been linked to obesity, heart disease, diabetes, cancer, and more. Even small quantities of as little as 1 to 2 grams of trans fats/day have been shown in studies to be dangerous. For comparison, if you eat a normal order of fries at a fast food joint or any restaurant, you can easily get 5 grams or more of trans fats. Now if as little as 1 gram daily can be dangerous to your health, imagine what you're doing to yourself with 5 grams…and that was only the fries! What about all of the cookies, cakes, chicken fingers, donuts, and other stuff people eat on a regular basis? Some people are getting more than 20-30 grams of trans fats every day and don't even realize that they're slowly killing themselves with this crap. If you care about your health, check the ingredients of everything you buy, and if you see partially hydrogenated oils of any kind, margarine, or shortening, protect yourself and your family by choosing something else. If I were asked to pick one thing that is most harmful to our health that is used in our food supply, it would be the artificial trans fats by a landslide. They are simply THAT dangerous that they must be avoided. In my opinion, artificial trans fats are right up there with cigarettes in terms of negative health effects. Because of the growing awareness and concern over the negative health effects of trans fats, the FDA mandated that all food manufacturers show the quantity of trans fat on all labels starting back in January 2006. However, they can still claim that their product is "trans fat free" or "no trans fat" if it has 0.5 grams of trans fat or less per serving according to regulations in the US. So all they have to do is reduce the serving size portion small enough so that it has 0.5 grams of trans, and they can claim "no trans fat". Don't trust them! You must inspect the ingredients for yourself to know if it's free of hydrogenated oils, margarine, or shortening.

- Refined oils: Even if the oils are not hydrogenated, most oils on your supermarket shelves are refined, even most of the so called "healthy" canola oils. Most refined oils still undergo the high temperature, high pressure, solvent extraction, bleaching, and deodorizing processes. Anything labeled vegetable oil, soybean oil, corn oil, cottonseed oil, safflower oil, and even many canola oils have been damaged by this refining process. This damages the natural structure of the fats, destroys natural antioxidants, creates free radicals, and produces a generally unhealthy product. Take note that the explosion of heart disease in the middle of the 20th century coincides quite nicely with the rapid increase in the use of hydrogenated and refined oils in the food supply at that time, while the consumption of **saturated fats has actually decreased** between the early 1900's and present time. Think about that. I think you'll begin to see the real culprit for heart disease…hydrogenated and refined oils, not the natural healthy saturated fats that have received an undeserved bad rap.

- Anything deep fried: including tortilla chips, potato chips, French fries, donuts, fried chicken, chicken nuggets, etc. It's all fried in hydrogenated or refined oils...most of the time using cheap oils like cottonseed or soybean oil. All of this crap doesn't even pass as real food in my opinion! If you can actually find something that's deep fried in a non-hydrogenated tropical oil like palm or coconut (which are stable oils under heat), then that might be the only deep fried food that's acceptable. It's unlikely you'll find that these days though.

- Homogenized milk fat - Milk fat is a very healthy fat in its natural raw state. Traditional populations around the world thrived in perfect health while consuming huge quantities of raw, non-pasteurized, non-homogenized, full fat dairy products. Once again, food processing ruins a good thing by pasteurizing and homogenizing milk fat, rendering it potentially dangerous inside the human body. Unfortunately, you will find it almost impossible to find raw milk in the US unless you personally know a farmer. Check out realmilk.com for more info on the benefits of raw milk and to find out if it's available near you. As an alternative, cultured dairy products like yogurt have at least had beneficial microorganisms added back to them making them better for you. Just watch out for the yogurts that are loaded with refined sugar and high fructose corn syrup. Instead, find one that's just lightly sweetened with honey or real maple syrup, or just use plain yogurt and add your own fruit to sweeten. Realistically, since you probably won't find raw milk, sticking to skim milk is probably the best option. Just keep in mind that a large percentage of the population has difficulty digesting (or has allergies to) cow's milk either due to the lactose for some people, and the proteins for others. If you use butter for cooking, cultured organic butter is the best option.

I hope this section has shed some light on the truth about dietary fats and made you realize their importance in a healthy diet. This doesn't mean I'm promoting any sort of gimmicky high-fat, low-carb diet. I'm simply trying to show you that a balanced diet including ample healthy fats (including the healthy saturated fats) is very important to your overall health and training results.

3.3 Healthy Trans Fats vs. Unhealthy Trans Fats Revealed

I'm going to talk about something in this section that most of you have probably never heard...that there is a distinction between good trans fats and bad trans fats. There is some evidence that the good trans can help you with fat loss, muscle building, and even cancer prevention, while the bad trans fats have been shown to cause heart disease, cancer, diabetes, and the general blubbering of your body.

I'm sure most of you have heard all of the ruckus in the news over the last few years about just how bad man-made trans fats are for your health. If you've been a reader of my newsletter and my "Truth about Six Pack Abs" e-book program, then you definitely know my opinion that these substances are some of the most evil food additives of all and are found in the vast majority of all processed foods and fast foods on the market today. In my opinion, man-made trans fats are right up there with smoking in terms of their degree of danger to your health. After all, they are one of THE MAIN factors for the explosion of heart disease since approximately the 1950's.

As you may have heard recently, the FDA has mandated that food manufacturers include the grams of trans fat on all nutrition labels starting back at the beginning of 2006. This means that as inventory is replaced in the grocery stores, you should start to see grams of trans listed on all packages from now on, providing you with an easier way to avoid them.

With all of the talk about trans fats in the news these days, I wanted to clarify some things, particularly regarding bad trans fats vs. good trans fats. If you've never heard of good trans fats before, let me explain in a bit.

The Bad Trans Fats
First, the bad trans fats I'm referring to are the man-made kind. These are represented by any artificially hydrogenated oils. The main culprits are margarine, shortening, and partially hydrogenated oils that are in most processed foods, junk

foods, and deep fried foods. These hydrogenated oils are highly processed using harsh chemical solvents like hexane (a component of gasoline), high heat, pressure, have a metal catalyst added, and are then deodorized and bleached. A small % of the solvent is allowed to remain in the finished oil. This has now become more of an industrial oil rather than a food oil, but somehow the FDA still allows the food manufacturers to put this crap in our food at huge quantities, even with the well documented health dangers.

These hydrogenated oils cause inflammation inside of your body, which signals the deposition of cholesterol as a healing agent on artery walls. Hence, hydrogenated oil = inflammation = clogged arteries. You can see why heart disease has exploded since this crap has been loaded into our food supply over the last 5 to 6 decades. As time goes on, and science continues to unveil how deadly these oils really are, I feel that eventually they will be illegal and banned from use. The labeling laws were just the first step. In fact, certain countries around the world have already banned the use of hydrogenated oils in food manufacturing or at least set dates to phase them out for good.

However, keep in mind that as companies are starting to phase out the use of hydrogenated oils in processed foods, they are replacing them, in most instances, with highly refined cheap vegetable oils. These are still heavily processed oils using high heat, solvents, deodorizers, and bleaching agents. Even refined oils are known to produce inflammation in your body...a far cry from natural sources of healthy fats. Once again, for the best results, your best bet is avoiding highly processed foods altogether and choose whole, natural, minimally processed foods. Your body will thank you!

The Good Trans Fats

Ok, after having trash talked the man-made trans fats, let me clearly state that there IS such a thing as healthy natural trans fats. Natural trans fats are created in the stomachs of ruminant animals like cattle, sheep, goats, etc. and make their way into the fat stores of the animals. Therefore, the milk fat and the fat within the meat of these animals can provide natural healthy trans fats. Natural trans fats in your diet have been thought to have some potential benefit to aid in both muscle building and fat loss efforts. However, keep in mind that the quantity of healthy trans fats in the meat and dairy of ruminant animals is greatly reduced by mass-production methods of farming and their grain and soy heavy diets. Meat and dairy from grass-fed, free-range animals always have much higher quantities of these beneficial fats.

One such natural trans fat that you may have heard of is called conjugated linoleic acid (CLA) and has been marketed by many weight loss companies. Keep in mind that these man-made CLA pills you see in the stores may not be the best way to get CLA in your diet. They are artificially made from plant oils, instead of the natural process that happens in ruminant animals. Once again, man-made just doesn't compare to the benefits of natural sources.

Now that all of your labels should be listing grams of trans fat, keep in mind that if a quantity of trans fat is listed on a meat or dairy product, it is most likely the natural good trans fats that we've discussed here. Otherwise, if the quantity of trans is listed on any processed foods, it is most likely the dangerous unhealthy crap from artificially hydrogenated oils, so stay away!

I hope you've enjoyed this interesting look at good trans fat vs. bad trans fat and use the info to arm yourself with more healthful food choices for a better body.

3.4 The Top Fitness Foods to Stock Your Cabinets With…Making Smart Choices Starts at the Grocery Store

In most of my newsletters, I like to provide a healthy snack or meal recipe that not only is delicious, but also helps to get you closer to that hard-body appearance that everyone is looking for. In this section, I'd like to give you healthy food ideas in a different way. This time, I figured I'd just give you some ideas of what I stock my kitchen with. Remember, if you don't have junk around the house, you're less likely to eat junk. If all you have is healthy food around the house, you're forced to make smart choices. Basically, it all starts with making smart choices and avoiding temptations when you make your grocery store trip. Now these are just some of my personal preferences, but perhaps they will give you some good ideas that you'll enjoy.

Alright, so let's start with the fridge. Each week, I try to make sure I'm loaded up with lots of varieties of fresh vegetables. During the growing season, I only get local produce, but obviously in winter, I have to resort to the produce at the grocery store. Most of the time, I make sure I have plenty of vegetables like zucchini, onions, asparagus, fresh mushrooms, spinach, broccoli, red peppers, etc. to use in my morning eggs. I also like to dice up some lean chicken or turkey sausage into the eggs, along with some swiss, jack, or goat cheeses. Coconut milk is another staple in my fridge. I like to use it to mix in with smoothies, oatmeal, or yogurt for a rich, creamy taste. Not only does coconut milk add a rich, creamy taste to lots of dishes, but it's also full of healthy saturated fats. Yeah, you heard me…I said healthy saturated fats! Healthy saturated fats like medium chain triglycerides, specifically an MCT called lauric acid. If the idea of healthy saturated fats is foreign to you, check out an eye-opening article at truthaboutabs.com called "The Truth about Saturated Fats".

Back to the fridge, some other staples:

• Cottage cheese, ricotta cheese, and yogurt - I like to mix cottage or ricotta cheese and yogurt together with chopped nuts and berries for a great mid-morning or mid-afternoon meal.

• Chopped walnuts, pecans, almonds, macadamias, etc. - delicious and great sources of healthy fats.

• Whole flax seeds - I grind these in a mini coffee grinder and add to yogurt or salads. Always grind them fresh because the omega-3 polyunsaturated fats are highly unstable and prone to oxidation, potentially creating inflammation causing free radicals from pre-ground flax.

• Whole eggs - one of natures richest sources of nutrients and high quality protein (and remember, they increase your GOOD cholesterol).

• Nut butters - Plain old peanut butter has gotten a little old for me, so I get creative and mix together almond butter with sesame seed butter, or even cashew butter with macadamia butter...delicious and unbeatable nutrition!

• Salsa - I try to get creative and try some of the exotic varieties of salsas.

• Butter - don't believe the naysayers; butter adds great flavor to anything and can be part of a healthy diet (just keep the quantity small because it is calorie dense...and NEVER use margarine, unless you want to assure yourself a heart attack).

• Avocados - love them...plus a great source of healthy fats, fiber, and other nutrients. Try adding them to wraps, salads, or sandwiches.

• Whole grain wraps and whole grain bread (look for wraps and bread with at least 3-4 grams of fiber per 20 grams of total carbs).

• Rice bran and wheat germ - these may sound way too healthy for some, but they actually add a nice little nutty, crunchy taste to yogurt or smoothies, or can be added when baking muffins or breads to add nutrients and fiber.

• Leaf lettuce and spinach along with shredded carrots - for salads with dinner.

• Home-made salad dressing - using balsamic vinegar, extra virgin olive oil, and Udo's Choice oil blend. This is much better than store bought salad dressing which mostly use highly refined soybean oil (source of inflammation-causing free radicals).

Some of the staples in the freezer:

• Frozen fish - I like to try a couple different kinds of fish each week. There are so many varieties out there, you never have to get bored. Plus, frozen fish is usually frozen immediately after catching, as opposed to fresh fish, which has been in transport and sitting at markets for days, allowing it more opportunity to spoil.

• Frozen berries - during the local growing season, I only get fresh berries, but during the other 10 months of the year, I always keep a supply of frozen blueberries, raspberries, blackberries, strawberries, cherries, etc. to add to high fiber cereal, oatmeal, cottage cheese, yogurt, or smoothies

• Frozen veggies - again, when the growing season is over and I can no longer get local fresh produce, frozen veggies are the best option, since they often have higher nutrient contents compared to the fresh produce that has been shipped thousands of miles, sitting around for weeks before making it to your dinner table.

• Frozen chicken breasts - very convenient to nuke up for a quick addition to wraps or chicken sandwiches for quick meals.

• Frozen buffalo, ostrich, venison, and other "exotic" lean meats – Yeah, I know, I'm weird, but I can tell you that these are some of the healthiest meats around, and if you're serious about a lean healthy body, these types of meats are much better for you than the mass produced, hormone-pumped beef and pork that's sold at most grocery stores.

Alright, now the staples in my cabinets:

• Oat bran and steel cut oats - higher fiber than those little packs of instant oats.

• Cans of coconut milk - to be transferred to a container in the fridge after opening.

• Various antioxidant rich teas - green, oolong, white, rooibos are some of the best. Surprisingly, even chammomile tea has been shown to provide important trace nutrients and antioxidants.

• Stevia - a natural non-caloric sweetener, which is an excellent alternative to the nasty chemical-laden artificial sweeteners like aspartame, saccharine, and sucralose.

• Organic maple syrup - none of that high fructose corn syrup Aunt Jemima crap...only real maple syrup can be considered real food. The only time I really use this (because of the high sugar load) is added to my post-workout smoothies to sweeten things up and also elicit an insulin surge to push nutrients into your muscles.

• Raw honey - better than processed honey...higher quantities of beneficial nutrients and enzymes. Honey has even been proven in studies to improve glucose metabolism (how you process carbs). I use a teaspoon or so every morning in my teas.

• Whole wheat or whole grain spelt pasta - much higher fiber than normal pastas

• Brown rice and other higher fiber rice - NEVER white rice

• Cans of black or kidney beans - I like to add a couple scoops to my Mexican wraps for the fiber and high nutrition content. Also, beans are surprisingly one of the best sources of youth promoting antioxidants!

• Tomato sauces - delicious, and as I'm sure you've heard a million times, they are a great source of lycopene. Just watch out for the brands that are loaded with nasty high fructose corn syrup.

• Dark chocolate (as dark as possible) - This is one of my treats that satisfies my sweet tooth, plus provides loads of antioxidants at the same time. It's still calorie dense, so I keep it to just a couple squares; but that is enough to do the trick, so I don't feel like I need to go out and get cake and ice cream to satisfy my dessert urges. Choose dark chocolate that lists it's cocoa content at 70% or greater. Milk chocolate is usually only about 30% cocoa, and even most cheap dark chocolates are only around 50% cocoa. Cocoa content is key for the antioxidant benefit...the rest is just sugar and other additives.

• Organic unsweetened cocoa powder - I like to mix this into my smoothies for an extra jolt of antioxidants or make my own low-sugar hot cocoa by mixing cocoa powder into hot milk with stevia and a couple melted dark chocolate chunks.

Of course, you also can never go wrong with any types of fresh fruits. Even though fruit contains natural sugars, the fiber within most fruits usually slows down the carbohydrate absorption and glycemic response. Also, you get the benefit of high antioxidant content and nutrient density in most fruits. Some of my favorites are kiwi, pomegranate, mango, papaya, grapes, oranges, fresh pineapple, bananas, apples, pears, peaches, and all types of berries.

Well, I hope you enjoyed this special look into my favorite lean body meals and how I stock my kitchen. Your tastes are probably quite different than mine, but hopefully this gave you some good ideas you can use next time you're at the grocery store looking to stock up a healthy and delicious pile of groceries.

3.5 Are Vitamin/Mineral Supplements Necessary or Just Money Down the Toilet?

As a fitness professional, I receive questions about vitamins all the time. Questions like......What kinds should I take? How much? Should I take a multi or just a couple of the important individual ones like C, E, calcium, or zinc? Will they help me lose weight or build muscle? So with all the talk and hype about vitamin and mineral supplements...Are they really necessary for optimal health? The answer is a definitive.....HELL NO! That is, if you're eating a balanced healthy diet, which most people don't. Let me put it this way...a vitamin/mineral supplement probably will be somewhat beneficial to you if you have a poor diet. However, if you're really serious about getting lean and ripped and truly healthy for good, why would your diet be poor? So, in the case that you're eating a healthy, balanced diet, the answer is that you don't need a vitamin supplement.

Let's think about this for a second. Did humans thrive on the planet for tens of thousands of years by popping an artificially created vitamin pill. Out of tens of thousands of years of human existence, vitamin pills have only been around for a couple of decades, yet the population is in worse health than ever before. Sure, maybe the human race is not in its worst health from a contagious disease perspective, but we definitely are from a degenerative disease perspective. Now I admit that we do live longer these days compared to historically, but that is only because medical advances keep us alive longer even though we are in horrendous shape physically. People might live longer now, but they're simply living longer while being overweight, crippled with degenerated joints, plagued with heart disease and cancers, and on and on. You get the point.

So let us get right to some answers as to why I contend that vitamin/mineral supplements are a waste of money and are not necessary to optimal health. Well, first and foremost, a healthy balanced diet consisting of a large variety of natural unprocessed foods (from meats, dairy, eggs, fruits, vegetables, grains, nuts, seeds, legumes, etc.) provides a rich array of vitamins, minerals, antioxidants, and all the other nutrients we need to thrive in perfect health. The problem is that many people don't choose a healthy balanced diet full of variety. They claim they are too busy, or it's too inconvenient. Well, I hope that you take your body and the health of you and your family more seriously than these people that apparently don't care about the physical being that they are walking around in day in and day out.

Another problem with attempting to obtain your vitamins and minerals from a pill instead of natural foods is that your body does not absorb and utilize the nutrients from a pill as efficiently as those obtained from natural food. Whole foods naturally contain vitamins and minerals in combinations that are best assimilated. On the other hand, vitamin/mineral pills contain lots of vitamins and minerals that many times interfere with each other. For example, zinc and copper taken at the same time interfere with each others absorption. Also, high doses of Vitamin E can interfere with absorption of beta carotene (a vitamin A precursor) and other fat soluble vitamins. Many other combinations interfere with each other as well.

Another problem with vitamin pills is possible excess consumption of fat soluble vitamins (vitamins A, D, E, and K). Fat soluble vitamins accumulate in fatty tissue in our bodies, and therefore it is easier to overdose on these compared with water soluble vitamins (vitamin C and the various B vitamins). Excess fat soluble vitamin accumulation can cause various toxic effects within the body. It is much harder to take in excess quantities of fat soluble vitamins through natural foods. You would have to consume exorbitant quantities of liver and other organ meats to take in too much Vitamin A and D. It would be rare for someone to overeat on foods such as that. Also, it would be hard to over consume a plant-based precursor to Vitamin A (beta carotene), found in sweet potatoes, carrots, etc., because your body simply would shut down the conversion to Vitamin A once it has obtained what it needs.

There are even some instances where mega-doses of water soluble vitamins can be toxic. Mega doses of some B vitamins can potentially cause nausea, vomiting, diarrhea, and even liver damage. However, in most instances, you simply excrete excess water soluble vitamins in your urine. That is why many times, your urine will be a deep yellow color a couple of hours after taking a vitamin that has high doses of vitamins B and C. So, when you take a vitamin pill, most of the water soluble vitamins are simply flushed down the toilet. You might as well just eliminate the middleman and flush your money right down the toilet!

Another problem with vitamin pills is that they often use synthetic versions of vitamins that can actually be unhealthy. For example, the forms of vitamin E that are found in pills can be either d-alpha tocopherol (a natural version) and dl-alpha tocopherol (a synthetic version). First of all, the bioavailability of synthetic vitamin E is much lower than natural vitamin E. In addition, I've seen many studies cited that indicated that there could be potential health dangers with taking synthetic vitamin E. Once again, we get back to the fact that natural is always better than something that has been heavily modified by man.

The bottom line is that as long as you eat a balanced diet full of a good variety of fruits, vegetables, nuts, seeds, whole grains, legumes, meats, dairy, eggs, etc., you will obtain all the nutrients your body needs to operate efficiently without the need for a manmade vitamin/mineral pill.

Exercise is obviously very important for losing body fat and building a strong, lean body, but always remember that proper nutrition is even more important. A lousy diet means a flabby, unhealthy body, regardless of how often someone works out.

3.6 Make Healthier Choices When Forced to Eat Fast-Food

I was out recently with some friends and we stopped at a fast food joint. I hate fast food joints, but sometimes when everybody else wants to go there, you just have to make the best of it and find something at least somewhat healthy. If you're forced to eat fast-food, here's a tip to make sure that you're not doing much damage to your body...ALWAYS AVOID the soda and anything deep fried including french fries, hash browns, and anything breaded like chicken nuggets, chicken patties, or breaded fish sandwiches. These are all absolutely soaked in deadly trans fats from the industrial hydrogenated vegetable oils they use to fry all of these items.

Remember, as I've said before, I've seen studies indicating that as little as 1-2 grams of trans fat per day can have serious degenerative internal effects in your body such as inflammation, clogging and hardening of the arteries, heart disease, various forms of cancer...not to mention packing on the ab flab. That's as little as 1-2 grams! Consider that a typical fast-food meal of a breaded chicken sandwich (or fish sandwich), along with an order of fries can contain as much as 10 grams of trans fat! Add on a cookie or small piece of pie for dessert (which are usually made with deadly margarine or shortening), and now you're up to about 13 grams of trans fat with that entire meal. If 1 gram a day is slowly killing you, imagine what 13 grams is doing! And that was only one meal that you ate. Some people are consuming 20-30 grams of trans fat per day, and not even realizing what they're doing to themselves internally. Please realize that nobody, I mean NOBODY, is looking out for your health, except for YOU.

Anyway, back to the topic of how to avoid this stuff and eat a reasonably healthy meal on the rare occasion that you're forced to eat fast-food. As for drinks, avoid the sodas...they're nothing but chemicals along with heavily processed high fructose corn syrup which will surely end up as extra belly blubber. Water is always the best drink, but if you need something with flavor, try unsweetened or lightly sweetened iced tea. At breakfast, the best choices are an egg, ham, and cheese on an english muffin (not on a croissant, which is full of nasty trans!), or one of those fruit & nut salads. At lunch or dinner, the best choices are a grilled chicken sandwich, the chili, a grilled chicken salad without croutons (again...croutons = more trans), or even just a plain cheeseburger. The main take-away point from this little fast-food article is that the nastiest stuff at these fast food joints are the sodas and fries, and any other deep fried items.

For any of you that have seen the movie "Super-Size Me", you saw how eating fast food every day absolutely destroyed that guy's health, but did you happen to notice the one guy that was the king of eating big macs (or some kind of burger)? I don't remember what kind of burger it was, but basically this guy has eaten these fast food burgers almost every day of his life for the past 30 years or something like that. Did you notice that he stated that he almost never eats the fries or soda, even though he eats the burgers every day? And he's not necessarily overweight. Now I'm not saying that fast-food burgers made with their refined white bread and low quality beef and cheese are the healthiest thing, but the point is...it's the fries and sodas that are the real health disaster.

Alright, so next time you're out at one of these places, remember these tips and choose smart!

By the way, if you haven't heard yet, McD's has started adding a nutrition label to all of their food wrappers, so now you can at least be aware what you're eating. Remember that as little as one gram of trans may cause some internal harm and now you can actually see how many grams of trans fat you're eating right on the food wrapper. That might change your mind about finishing it.

Well, I hope you've enjoyed this book. I tried to give you some of my insider secrets of a fitness junkie for developing a lean, muscular, and truly healthy body for life!